Organic Natural Antibiotics And Antivirals For Beginners

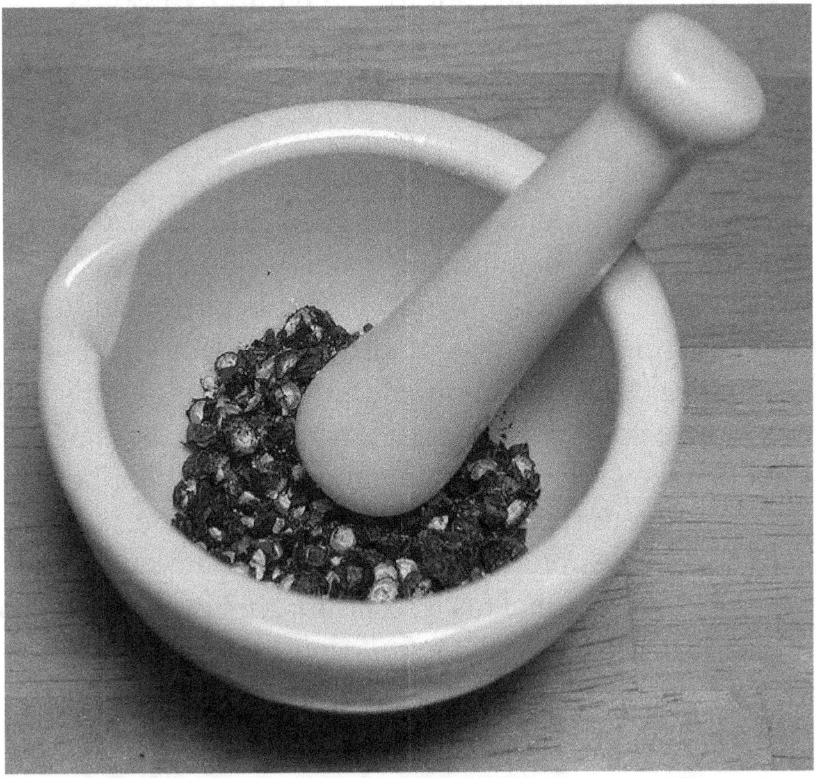

How To Use Homemade, Medicinal Herbs To Prevent Illness And Infectious Diseases

By Dr Alex Nelson

Disclaimer

This book is intended to be a general guide, to raise awareness, and to help people make informed decisions in the context of their own personal circumstance. As everybody's circumstances are different, so are the remedies you should seek. While many of the recommendations in this book can be applied by almost anybody regardless of their conditions they are not intended to and should not be relied upon to replace personal medical advice.

The author accepts no responsibility for any loss or injury, be it personal or financial, as a result for the use or misuse of the information in this book. If you have any doubts or concerns after reading this book, please speak to a doctor or other qualified person before taking any actions.

Contents

Introduction

Chapter 1
An Overview Of Antibiotics And Antivirals

Chapter 2
The Pros And Cons Of Synthetic Antibiotics

Chapter 3
How You Can Benefit From Using Natural Antibiotics And Antivirals

Chapter 4
10 Herbs That Antibiotic Herbs And Antiviral Properties

Chapter 5
Foods That Have Natural Antibiotic And Antiviral Properties

Introduction

Our bodies are equipped with a built-in protection system, called the immune system that defends us from nasty and health-threatening bacteria and viruses. Our immune system is amazingly crafted giving us the power and the capability to protect ourselves from internal threats, which may not be noticed by our naked eyes. Whenever we get hit by bad bacteria and harmful viruses our immune system acts either as our army and attacks these foreign invaders or as some kind of wall and stop them from spreading throughout our bodies.

However, our protection wall and our army are not always strong enough to battle the harmful bacteria and viruses. Some of them are too sophisticated for our built-in protection to handle. Also sometimes, because of our unhealthy lifestyle and the amount of stressors that we are exposed to every single day, our immune systems and resistance to pathogens go down and become weak to fight these bacteria and viruses. When these circumstances happen, we already need to turn to the aid of antibiotics and antivirals to back our immune systems up and help fight these invaders.

Now, the question is: *What exactly are antibiotics and antivirals and what are their differences or similarities?* This ebook will answer these questions and at the same time discuss relevant topics that are concerned with antibacterial and antivirals and with their uses.

Chapter 1 is an overview about antibiotics and antivirals. The difference between the two will be explained, as well as their specific uses.

Chapter 2 will tackle on the advantages and the disadvantages of using synthetic antibiotics.

The benefits of using natural antibiotics and antivirals will be explained in Chapter 3. You will know the comparative effects of natural substances versus synthetic ones.

Chapters 4, 5 and 6 will enumerate some of the herbs, foods and oils that have natural antimicrobial properties.

And lastly, Chapter 7 will give you tips and recipes on how to craft your own natural antivirals and antibiotics right at the vicinity of your own kitchen.

Chapter 1
An Overview Of Antibiotics And Antivirals

Antibiotics and antivirals help our bodies fight foreign organisms especially when our immune system is too weak to fight these organisms. They serve as back up or substitute fighters at times when our built-in protection cannot fight back.

So, what really are similarities and difference of these so-called antibiotics and antivirals? When can we use an antibiotic or antivirals? This chapter will answer frequently asked questions about them as well as provide an in depth information about their uses and correct your preconceived notions about these substances.

Virus VS Bacteria

Before we discover the similarities and the differences between antivirals and antibiotics, it is imperative that we know first the difference between a virus and a bacterium because the distinction of the two paves the way to the understanding of the difference of antivirals and antibiotics. Identifying whether an infection has been caused by a virus or bacteria is the key to knowing whether which kind of antimicrobial substance is more appropriate to use, antiviral or antibiotics.

Both bacteria and virus often cause infections that have almost the same symptoms, making it difficult to determine which of the two really caused the illness or disease. They also both have the ability to mutate and build resistance against antivirals and antibacterials, making them serious forces to be reckoned with.

However, the difference between bacteria and a virus lies in the absence or presence of a host. Bacteria are microorganisms that are ubiquitous and can adapt to any environment in order for it to survive. Although some bacteria are detrimental to one's health, good bacteria also exist and they are mainly present in the intestines as aid for digestion. Viruses, on the other hand, are smaller microorganisms and depend on a host for its survival. There is a cessation in the growth of viruses when they have no host to feed on. Unlike bacteria, viruses cannot reproduce. Instead, they mess up the mechanism of the cells and dictate them to produce the virus. Compared to bacteria, viruses develop resistance to antimicrobials faster. Bacteria may build resistance after a month or a year but viruses develop resistance and mutate as rapidly as a day or a week after.

Viruses cause diseases such as colds and flu while bacteria cause wound infections.

Antibiotics

The word **"antibiotics"** came from the Greek words "**anti**", which means opposed to or against, and "**bios**", which means life. Basically, "*antibiotics*" means "*against life or opposed to life*". To be more scientific and specific, an antibiotic is a substance that either fights bacterial infections and kills them or prevents the reproduction or growth of the bacteria that are causing the infection and impede them from multiplying. This substance originates from a microorganism, which control the spread of bacteria or exterminate other bacteria.

Antibiotics are also commonly known as antibacterials because their main purpose is to fight infections that are caused by bacteria, not by viruses. Almost all antibiotics are not used to cure infections brought about by viruses and it must be emphasized that antibiotics do not cure and are not effective in treating viral infections.

The History of Antibiotics

The history of the use of antibiotics can be traced way back in the ancient civilizations. People utilized plants and other natural concoctions to treat their wounds, bites and other infections. For example, moulds from bread were used as treatment for wounds by the ancient people of Greece and the Chinese also utilized different kinds of herbs to treat infections. These just go to show that the use of antibiotics to treat infections is not a recent discovery in the field of medicine.

Although ancient people already used natural antibiotics, they most probably didn't know the science behind it. The people in the modern age provided the missing information about bacteria and antibiotics that the ancient people failed to give. Modern Age scientists treated bacteria more scientifically and logically and numerous names surfaced and became popular because of their relevant contributions in the field of microbiology and bacteriology. One of these names is the name of Alexander Fleming.

Sir Alexander Fleming invented the Penicillin, the world's first and most popular antibiotic, in the year 1928. This invention was an honest coincidence and a serendipitous discovery but it was such a great discovery that opened new doors in the field. It was a great stepping-stone to the formulation of modern antibiotics.

Classifications Of Antibiotics

Antibiotics are commonly classified according to the range of organisms that they can target, its way of administration, and their function.

In terms of the range of organisms that they can target, a certain kind of antibiotic can be classified as broad-spectrum or narrow-spectrum. Broad-spectrum antibiotics, just like the Fluoroquinolones, only means that these kinds of antibiotics can target a wide range of bacteria and other microorganisms and can treat several kinds of bacterial infections. The narrow-spectrum antibiotics can cure only a lesser number of bacterial infections compared to the broad-spectrum antibiotics.

Antibiotics are also classified according to the way they are taken in. They can be taken orally, meaning they are ingested in the form of capsules or syrups; topically, meaning they are applied as lotions or creams or ointments directly to the affected body parts; or through injection, which means you have to infuse the antibiotics to your systems. Topical antibiotics are usually used as treatment for skin infections while injectable antibiotics are used for more serious bacterial infections.

Lastly, antibiotics are also grouped according to what they can do. Antibiotics can either be bactericidal, meaning their purpose is to kill and impede the bacteria's cell wall from forming; or they could be bacteriostatic which means that these kinds of antibiotics will stop bacteria from growing in numbers. An example of a bactericidal antibiotic is Penicillin and examples of bacteriostatic antibiotics are tetracyclines.

Types Of Antibiotics

Here are some of the common types of antibiotics and their respective uses:

Penicillin
- These are used for a wide variety of bacterial infection including bacterial infections in the urinary tract.

Aminoglycosides

- Aminoglycosides are among the very powerful antibiotics which must be taken carefully and with proper prescription because it can cause serious injury such as damaged kidneys and loss of hearing when taken in high dosage.

- Since this kind of antibiotic breaks down easily, it is given through injections.

Fluoroquinolones

- This antibiotic belongs to the broad-spectrum antibiotics and can cure a wide range if infections.

- An example of this antibiotic is Cipro.

Maerolides

- This is a good alternative to penicillin and can treat infections in the lungs and chest area.

Tetracyclides

- Tetracyclides can be used as treatment for severe acne.

Caphalosporins

- This is effective in the treatment of serious infections such as meningitis.

Common Bacterial Infections

Some of the most common infections that people get from bacteria are salmonella, tuberculosis, syphilis, meningitis, strep throat, urinary tract infections, respiratory infections, boils, pneumonia and acne. Bacterial infections differ in the levels of threat that they inflict on humans and their threat basically depends on the kind of bacteria. We don't need to be too worried about some of the bacterial infections, such as acne or strep throat or boils. However, we must seek immediate treatment should we acquire bacterial infections such as meningitis or tuberculosis or syphilis because these infections can be life threatening.

Antivirals

The virus that targets the body and the one that targets the computer system operate in the same manner. The virus in the body makes us their host and causes a disorientation to our cellular processes in the same way that the virus in our computers feeds on the hardware or the software and mess up the normal process of the computer.

The word "**virus**" comes from the Latin word "**vīrus**" which means poison so the term "**antiviral**" literally means "against poison". By scientific definition, antivirals are medications that can fight infectious diseases caused by viruses. They treat infections either by stopping or slowing down the reproduction of the viruses in our system or by boosting the power of our immune system to fight the virus. The power of antivirals are only limited to inhibiting the growth of the virus and stop it from growing and reproducing. They cannot fully kill or exterminate the virus, unlike what the antibiotics can do.

Antivirals are utilized for the treatment of a relatively small range of organisms and there are different varieties of antiviral treatment for a specific kind of infections. They are also used in two ways, either as vaccines or as treatments to infections. As vaccines, antivirals serve as precaution and they prevent infections from developing. When used as treatment, antivirals can reduce the length of time that the symptoms of the infections are felt by a person. In other words, they lessen the damage that the virus causes.

Common Viral Infections

Like bacterial infections, viral infections are also placed in a continuum, depending on the level of harm that they can cause to our bodies. Some viral infections can be treated at once but some can cause extreme consequences such as death.

The common viral infections that are suffered by millions of people include colds, flu and other sophisticated strains of influenza such as the swine flu or the H1N1, hepatitis, sexually transmitted infections such as HIV or Human Immunodeficiency Virus, AIDS or Acquired Immune Deficiency Syndrome, herpes, and now, the dreaded Ebola virus infection.

Antibiotic VS Antivirals

The definitions of antibiotic and antiviral, as well as their uses have already been tackled in the previous paragraphs. At this juncture, the two will be contrasted and compared side by side in order to foster a better understanding about the two and a clearer distinction between them.

Similarities

Antivirals and antibiotics are similar on three grounds: (a) they both target the microorganism that is causing the infection, (b) they are both kinds of antimicrobials, which mean they can either destruct the microorganism or they can inhibit its growth, (c) and they both can be taken in various ways such as oral, topical or through injection.

Differences

There are clear differences between antibiotics and antimicrobials too even if they are both under the classification of antimicrobial substances. For starters, antibiotics are for bacterial infections while antivirals are for viral infections. Antibiotics cannot also treat infections caused by viruses. Unlike antibacterials that can kill the microorganisms and stop the bacteria from growing, antivirals cannot destroy viruses and they can only inhibit the growth of the virus. Also, antivirals are much more difficult to develop than antibacterials for the reason that killing the virus can also mean damaging the cells of the host. Another difference between the two is that antibiotics can be used to treat a wide range of infections while antivirals can treat more specific infections.

Chapter 2
The Pros And Cons Of Synthetic Antibiotics

There are a lot of aspects of our day-to-day lives that developed together with the innovation of modern technology. One of these aspects is the way we attend to diseases and illnesses. The discovery of modern medical apparatuses paved the way to the discovery of modern drugs and cures for a new generation of bacteria and viruses. Antibiotics, which were formulated in medical laboratories, replaced natural antibiotics and the once popular Penicillin became somewhat obsolete with the formulation of new synthetic antibiotics.

The synthetic antibiotics rose to fame after Penicillin was observed to be a major cause of allergic reaction to a majority of people and after it failed to cure new kinds of bacteria. Synthetic antibiotics, such as the Amoxicillin became the alternative for Penicillin because it is cheaper, more affordable and more effective.

However, not only the advantages of these synthetic drugs were discovered as they became largely available to the market. Hidden disadvantages that were lurking behind the effectiveness of these synthetic drugs were also discovered. This chapter is devoted to the discussion of the pros and cons of these synthetic drugs.

Pros of Synthetic Antibiotics

The reason that synthetic antibiotics still thrive in the market despite their side effects is because they are very effective. Synthetically produced antibiotics can effectively kill bacteria that are causing the infection. They work and diminish the bacteria fast and they do it efficaciously. In times of great need and in times of emergencies, these synthetic antibacterials can really help avert infection and help save a life.

Cons of Synthetic Antibiotics
One of the most serious side effects of synthetic antibiotics is bacterial resistance. This is a phenomenon whereby the bacteria that a specific kind of antibiotic is supposed to cure become resistant or somewhat immune to that kind of antibiotic. The bacteria then mutate and evolve and become stronger than the antibiotic itself. This happens because most people are abusing the use of and misusing antibiotics. Most of us are guilty of not giving our immune system the chance to fight the bacteria and just being dependent upon antibiotics even if the infection is not that serious. Another reason why bacteria become resistant to certain antibiotics is because we sometimes don't finish taking our prescriptions. I know that a lot of people are guilty of this. We have the tendency to stop taking the antibiotic drugs given to us once we feel better even if we were advised to take them longer. There is a reason why antibiotics are prescribed to be taken for a specific number of days and that is to make sure that the drug kills all of the bacteria. Cutting our medication short can foster the growth of a stronger kind of bacteria that are much harder to cure than their previous kind. These kinds of bacteria cause worse infections that, if not treated, are much longer to kill.

Another disadvantage of synthetic antibiotics is that they are toxic and they can introduce toxins to our systems. These toxins that synthetic antibiotics carry with them inside our bodies can cause our immune systems to weaken, causing it to fail in protecting us from the threat of these bacteria and consequently, making us more vulnerable to bacterial infections.

In addition to these side effects, synthetic antibiotics, due to their powerful and effective ability to kill off bacteria, can also accidentally kill off the healthy bacteria that live in our intestine. These innocent bacteria, which cause us wellness than harm and aid in our digestion, get accidentally killed together with the harmful and bad bacteria. This leads to intestinal problems like diarrhoea and indigestion.

Some of the other side effects of antibiotics are kidney stones, vomiting, allergic reactions especially to Penicillin and Cephalosporin, chronic fatigue syndrome and deafness. Yes you read that right. Some antibiotics are also ototoxic drugs, which means that they can cause damage to the cochlea or the vestibular system. High dosages of some powerful antibiotics like the Aminoglycosides can cause damage to the vestibular system. There was even this popular case of a woman who felt like she was perpetually falling because she was given high dosages of Gentamicin, a kind of antibiotic. The constant use of Gentamicin damaged the structures of her inner ear that are responsible for giving her sense of balance.

And the most important disadvantage in using synthetic antibiotics is that it is harmful to the environment. Since they are synthetic, which means they are made out of mixing chemicals, they have the potential to pollute the environment due to the by-products and waste materials that are produced out of mixing these chemicals.

Precautionary Measures To Consider Before Taking Antibiotics

Synthetic antibiotics should really be given and used properly, responsibly and wisely. Although they are highly effective in treating bacterial infections, they must be taken with some precautionary measures in order to avoid their harmful side effects. First, you must give your body the chance to fight certain bacteria before turning to antibiotics for help because we have natural bacteria fighters. We must use our built in power to fight bacterial infections in order to make us less vulnerable to the bacteria that cause these infections. Second, make sure that you consult your physician first before taking any kind of antibiotic. You must know what kind of bacterial infection you have and you must not take other people's prescriptions. Third, you must finish taking your prescription up to the last day that the doctor instructed in order to prevent bacteria from becoming resistant to the drug and to prevent the formation of super bacteria. Lastly, you must consider your tolerance to a specific kind of antibiotic. Make sure that you will not have allergic reactions to these antibiotics and you must also make sure that you are not pregnant because some antibiotics can cause birth defects and spontaneous abortions.

Chapter 3
How You Can Benefit From Using Natural Antibiotics And Antivirals

The previous chapter discussed the advantages and disadvantages of synthetic antibiotics and it was pretty clear that they could cause a lot of side effects, most of which are detrimental to our health. So why, despite the clear evidence that the disadvantages outweigh the advantages of using synthetic antibiotics, do people still use them? The answer to that is maybe because people don't trust the natural counterparts of synthetic antibiotics enough to make them start using them as alternative. Another reason could be the high effectiveness of these synthetic antibiotics. Or maybe, most people don't realize that there are natural alternative in the first place. This chapter is dedicated to the discussion of the benefits that you can reap out of using natural antibiotics and antivirals.

Natural Antibiotics and Antivirals
Yes. Natural antibiotics and antivirals do exist. In fact, their effects are much more powerful than synthetic antimicrobials. Not only do they help boost our immune system and help us be more resistant to infections, they can also serve as anti-inflammatory agents that stop the spread of infection and cause acceleration of the healing process.

Synthetic Antimicrobials VS Natural Antivirals and Antibiotics

Both synthetic and natural antivirals and antibiotics are effective in treating infections caused by bacteria or viruses. The only difference between the two is that synthetic antivirals and antibiotics are produced from mixing different chemicals in a laboratory to achieve the antibacterial properties of natural antimicrobials. On the other hand, natural antivirals and antibiotics are not produced in a lab and they are just produced from natural ingredients, which are present in plants.

Although both synthetic and natural antivirals and antibiotics can kill good bacteria, natural antimicrobials lesser good bacteria compared to synthetic alternatives.

Benefits of Using Natural Antivirals and Antibiotics

So what really are the benefits of natural antimicrobials? There are absolutely many! For starters, we don't have to worry about harmful toxins that enter our systems together with the antibiotics or antivirals that we ingest since they are made from plants and herbs. Also, the usage of the natural cures makes it harder for bacteria and viruses to be resistant to them. This is because natural antivirals and antibiotics have more compounds unlike synthetically produced antimicrobials, which come from only one compound. These numerous compounds present in plants cooperate with one another in making a strong antibiotic or antiviral substance that most bacteria and viruses have difficulty surviving from. Most herbal remedies to bacterial and viral infections are also cheaper compared to artificially produced antibiotics and antivirals. Also, most of the herbs that have antiviral or antibacterial properties are common in our surroundings and are generally accessible to us. And the most important benefit that can be derived from the usage of natural antivirals and antibiotics is that they are do not pollute the environment. These herbal cures are not derived from harmful chemicals that can pollute the environment so using them is more environment-friendly.

There really are a lot of advantages in using natural remedies to viral and bacterial infections. Maybe it is time that we appreciate them and convert to the use of plant-based or natural cures.

Chapter 4
10 Herbs That Antibiotic Herbs And Antiviral Properties

The reason why natural remedies to infections caused by bacteria or viruses are called "natural" is because they can be found in nature or they are present in the environment. They can be in plants or herbs or fruits or even in leaves and flowers. Whoever or whatever made us really provided us with an environment filled with everything that we could possibly need.

Although there are only a relatively few number of herbs that have antimicrobial properties, they are widely common anyway so as far as accessibility to these plants is concerned, we don't have to really worry.

In this chapter, the top 10 herbs that have antiviral or antibacterial properties will be listed as well as the illnesses and diseases that they can cure (5 herbs with antibiotic properties and 5 herbs that have antiviral properties). Find out whether the herbs that will be mentioned are present in your garden or available in your local grocery store.

Herbs That Have Antibacterial Properties

Calendula
Calendulas are also commonly known as pot marigold. Its small yellow or orange flowers are used as first aid treatment to wounds and infections. It is also a known cure for acute conjunctivitis or what is commonly known as pinkeye.

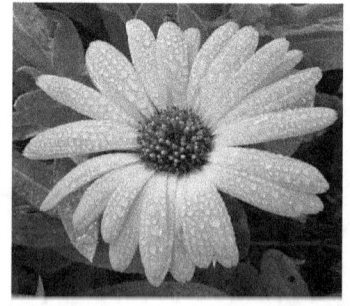

Cinnamon

Little do we know, cinnamon have antibacterial properties too and they are not just added to our coffees or to our bread. Cinnamon has antibacterial properties that can help in digestion. It is also a carminative, which means that taking it can help us pass gas or fart.

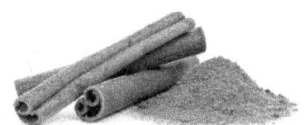

Yarrow

Yarrows are plants that have leaves resembling that of the fern and have whitish or yellowish flowers. Its powdered flowers, when mixed with water, are used to treat sores. They can also quickly stop wounds from bleeding and can also cure urinary tract infections.

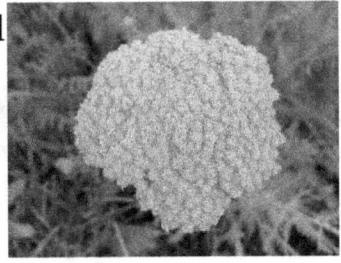

Garlic

Believe it or not, garlic is actually more effective in treating bacterial infections than Sir Fleming's Penicillin. It owes its antibacterial properties to the compound called allicin. Garlic is used as a first aid treatment for bites, especially dog bites and wounds.

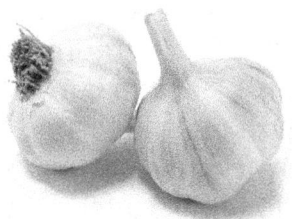

Aloe vera

Aloe vera has been proven to be very effective in treating burns because of its cooling effect. It can also prevent infections and can boost up the healing of wounds.

Actually, aloe vera has an antiviral property too and it can even cure simple herpes virus.

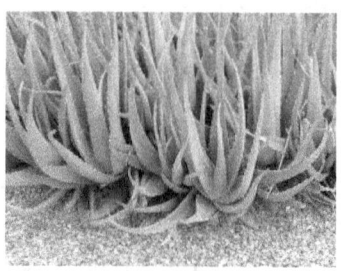

Herb That Have Antiviral Properties

Ginger

Ginger does not only make your voice sound more wonderful but it can also treat common colds and cough. Most people take ginger in the form of tea or in capsules.

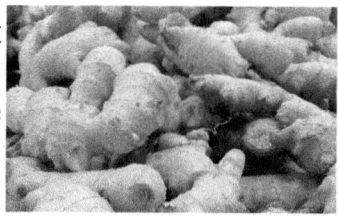

Olive leaf

Colds, flu and herpes are just a few of the viral infections that the olive leaf can cure. It can be taken orally in the form of tea or capsules. Expectant mothers should avoid this though because it can cause problems for pregnant women.

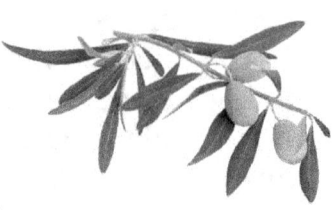

Oregano

The oregano belongs to the family of mints and gives off an aromatic odour. It is commonly used as spice or seasoning but it has antiviral properties as well. It can cure cough and common colds.

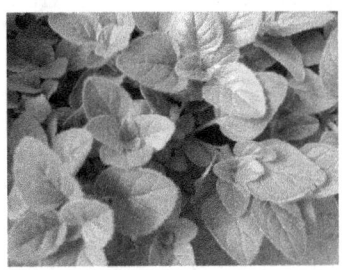

Cranberry

Almost everyone loves cranberry juice. Well, you will love it more for sure because it has antiviral properties and it is an antioxidant as well. Cranberry is used as treatment for urinary tract infections and it also keeps your teeth strong by preventing the formation of plaque.

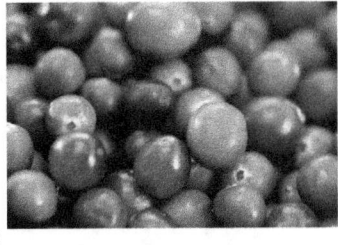

Cat's claw

Cat's claw helps us become less vulnerable to viral infections by making our immune system stronger. It also has anti-fungal and antibacterial properties.

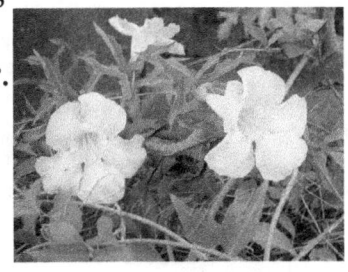

Actually, there are a lot more plants and herbs that have antibacterial and/or antiviral properties. There are also some, which may have these properties, but there are no exhaustive studies about their healing potentials yet. Hopefully, more scientists and doctors would be more open to natural medicines and research on the medicinal properties of some plants in order to fully utilize nature's potential and in order for us to finally let go of these harmful synthetic medicines.

Chapter 5
Foods That Have Natural Antibiotic And Antiviral Properties

Of course, all of us need to eat. We get most of our energy, as well as the essential nutrients and vitamins that our body needs from the food that we eat. This is the reason why it is important that we should eat healthy as often as possible and try to munch on green leafy vegetables and juicy fruits instead of junk foods. Another thing that can entice us to eat healthy is the fact that there are certain foods that can help us build a stronger immune system and help us fight viral and bacterial infections.

This chapter will tell you what kinds of food have the ability to fight harmful bacteria and viruses and as you read along, try to see if you have been partaking these foods lately.

Fruits Rich In Vitamin C

Fruits such as pineapples, oranges, lemons, strawberries and watermelon, as well as vegetables such as cabbage, cauliflower and broccoli are rich in Vitamin C. This vitamin keeps our immune systems strong and formidable against the threat of viruses and bacteria, therefore making us more resistant to harmful infections.

Stocking up in Vitamin C and eating foods that contain Vitamin C can help treat and prevent colds, cough, and skin infections.

Coconut

Coconut is considered is the wonder fruit because all of its parts, from top to bottom, have a relevant use to humans. The coconut fruit has medium-chain fatty acids that can destroy pathogens and can battle viruses and bacteria.

Breast Milk

There is a reason why they say that breast milk is the best for babies. It is because it has antibacterial and antiviral properties aside from the nutrients, minerals and vitamins that it contains. The immune systems of babies are not as strong as those of older individuals. That is why mothers should breast feed their babies in order to give them the necessary protection from infectious diseases.

The human breast milk is an abundant source of lauric acid, a medium-chain fatty acid that kills pathogens. The lauric acid helps in building a strong immune system that is more resistant to viruses and bacteria. That is probably the reason why breast-fed babies don't get easily infected by viruses and bacteria compared to babies who are not.

Yoghurt

Yoghurts and other prebiotics increase the number of good bacteria living in the intestines and help make digestion smoother and easier. This ability helps fight off infections and helps kill the unwanted invaders such as viruses and bacteria.

So, are you keeping your immune system strong by eating these foods?

Chapter 6
Essential Oils That Have Natural Natural Antibiotic And Antiviral Properties

We are already done discussing herbs and foods that have natural antiviral and antibiotic properties. Now it is time to know what are some of the oils that possess these properties too.

This chapter will discuss the examples of oils that either have cure viral infections or bacterial infections or both. The specific diseases and ailments that they can cure will also be tackled.

Eucalyptus Essential Oil
Eucalyptus, which has insecticidal, antibacterial and anti-inflammatory properties, works perfectly with coughs, colds and irritations. It is even a common component or ingredient in rubs and ointments.

Lemon Essential Oil
Lemon is popularly known for its antiseptic powers. It can cleanse wounds and prevent infections as well as make the healing process faster. Lemon oil is also a good antioxidant and helps the body get rid of all the harmful toxins. It can also be used applied directly to the skin as cleanser or wound antiseptic.

Peppermint Essential Oil
Peppermint oil has a wide variety of uses. It can be utilized as an antiseptic, antibacterial, antiviral and even anti-inflammatory. It can cure nausea and other digestive diseases.

Virgin Coconut Oil

The oil extracted from heating coconut water can have a lot of health benefits. It can cure mouth infections, aid in digestion, heal wounds and help moisturise irritated and dry skin.

Chapter 7
How To Prepare And Use Natural Antibiotics And Antivirals

At this juncture, you are probably enticed already to use antivirals and antibiotics that can naturally be found around us because of the all the benefits of these natural antimicrobials and their availability. If you are, then it is very good that you are opening your doors for herbal cures and have considered using them instead of the artificially made ones.

So, the next question that you might be probably thinking in your head is this: *How do I use these natural antibiotics and antivirals?* The answer simple: Natural antivirals and antibiotics, just like synthetic antimicrobials, can be taken orally or topically, which means they can used as capsules, ointments, rubs or drinks. You have to be careful though and take into consideration a few things, just like your skin sensitivity to the natural treatment, which are applied topically. You must also take into consideration whether or not you are pregnant by the time you want to take these natural cured because some of them are harmful to pregnant women. You also need to have sufficient knowledge about the natural treatment that you want to take because some of them need to be diluted because of their strong effects.

This chapter will teach you to prepare natural antivirals and antibiotics as well as some natural remedies to skin problems and common ailments.

Preparing Natural Antivirals And Antibiotics

These are some simple and comprehensive steps on

how to prepare natural antimicrobials.

Natural Ointments

To make antiviral ointments, you must mix a maximum of 4 drops of one or more kinds of antiviral oils into pure coconut oil. Store in a glass jar and keep away from the reach of small children.

You can also utilize aloe vera as an ointment for burns. You can heat some aloe vera leaves before slicing them or you can slice them right away. Make sure that the transparent and colourless gooey substance is applied thoroughly throughout the burnt area.

Natural Cough Treatment

You can add mint leaves or Oregano leaves to a pot of water and boil it for 10 to 20 minutes. When the water becomes greenish or when you can already smell the aroma of the oregano or the mint mixing with the water, you can already drink the concoction.

Tea

To make your own herbal tea, all you need is a cup of hot water and any antiviral or antibacterial herb of your choice. Mix 1 tablespoon of antimicrobial herbs into a cup of water and leave it for 5 to 10 minutes. Drink when ready.

5 Natural Remedies For Common Ailments

It is important that we know some first aid treatments to common ailments because knowing such information can help save a life and prevent the spread of infection.

Here are 5 of the most common ailments acquired by most people and their natural cures:

1. _Colds_

Getting a cold is one manifestation of a down immune system. It is your body's way of telling you that your natural defences are weak. The natural ways of treating colds is by drinking lots and lots of water to flush out the toxins in your body or by drinking tea with ginger. You can also opt for an overdose of Vitamin C through eating a lot of fruits rich in Vitamin C. You don't have to worry about overdosing in Vitamin C because it is water-soluble and the body can easily get rid of the excess Vitamin C in our system by urinating.

2. _Stomach Ache_

Drinking chamomile tea, or hot water with ginger or peppermint can help in indigestion.

3. _Burns_

For less serious burns, aloe vera can be used to cool off the burnt part of the skin. If ever the burn is already a second-degree burn, go immediately to the hospital and let the doctors handle it.

4. _Wounds_

A lot of herbs can be used to treat wounds and prevent them from getting infected. You can use lemon juice to clean the wound and to disinfect it. Warning: This may be very painful. You can also use garlic.

5. *Flu*

- Flu can be cured by the help of drinking lots of fluids and eating vegetables and fruits rich in Vitamin C.

5 Natural Skin Care Remedies

Taking good care of the skin is important, especially for the ladies. Fortunately, nature also offers skin remedies that help us cure common skin diseases that are very stubborn to cure. There are also natural substances that can help us keep our skin young and glowing. Here are some of them:

1. *Sugar mixed with coconut oil*

- Does your skin appear dull and old? There's need to worry because nature has a solution for you! This mixture can serve as the natural equivalent to exfoliators. It can exfoliate dead skin cells, resulting to a softer and younger skin.

2. *Vitamin C*

- Vitamin C can help the skin become more youthful and firmer by facilitating the production of collagen to repair damaged cells.

3. *Honey mixed with water*

- This mixture serves as a perfect facial mask which helps cleanse the face and get rid of the excess oil and dirt.

4. _Coconut oil_

- Coconut oil can help moisturize the skin and keep it smooth and silky. It also prevents skin irritations.

5. _Oatmeal_

- Oatmeal can actually cure inflammations and tone down allergic reactions.

Conclusion

I hope that you have learned a lot about antibiotics and antivirals after reading this ebook. I also hope that you will apply your new found knowledge about these antimicrobials into good use and encourage others to discover the benefits of natural treatments such as herbal antivirals and antibiotics, oils, as well as the foods that have and contain these antimicrobial properties.

I would also like to reiterate the importance of the body's natural defence system in fighting against these invaders. Just once again emphasize the point, we must allow our bodies to fight these harmful bacteria and viruses because we have the capability to do so. Impeding this capability can cause our defences to weaken and makes us more vulnerable to these invaders. Also, we must not allow ourselves to be dependent to these antimicrobials because some of them, especially the synthetically produced ones, have harmful effects on the body.

The herbs, oils, foods and other natural treatments stated in this ebook are not the only ones that have antimicrobial properties. There are still a lot of plants that also have the ability to fight off these harmful invaders waiting to be discovered.

Lastly, I hope that more researches about the effectiveness of natural treatment against harmful bacteria and viruses will surface in the medical industry and promote the use of natural cures instead of the synthetic ones.

From The Author

Thank you for taking the time to read this book. As an author, I understand the importance of creating books which my readers will find both enjoyable and informative. If you have the time and feel generous, please don't hesitate to leave an honest review of this book.........*Dr Alex Nelson.*

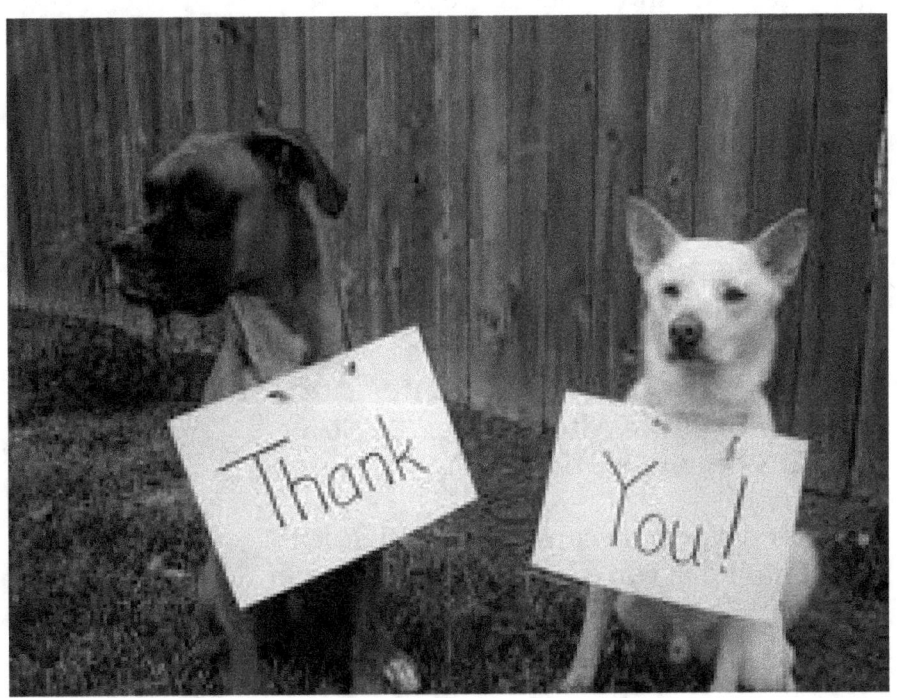

Other Books By Dr Alex Nelson

Cure Adrenal Fatigue Now!

Adrenal Fatigue doesn't have to control your life. There are solutions to help you diagnose and overcome this modern day symptom of stress. Within the pages of this easy-to-read guide, Dr. Alex Nelson, has outlined all the information you need to know in order to combat the dreaded listlessness and show you the steps necessary to recharge your energy levels and leave you feeling invigorated and ready for any of life's challenges. Discover the natural remedies that can and will change your life.

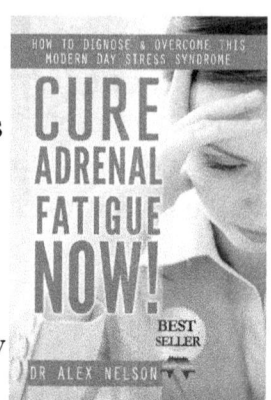

Natural Remedies For Beginners

Are You Looking For Healthier And More Affordable Alternatives To Store Bought Pharmaceuticals?

Day after day, we are constantly bombarded with stimuli that can cause harmful effects on our bodies just like a stressful job, a highly competitive group of classmates, a messy family, a demanding lover and even terror bosses and teachers. Pair those with a polluted environment and keeping an unhealthy lifestyle, it is really possible that we sometimes lose the battle to sickness. We can get infections and diseases that can rob our energy away from us and even force us to stay in bed. However, with the rise in the prices of medicine and

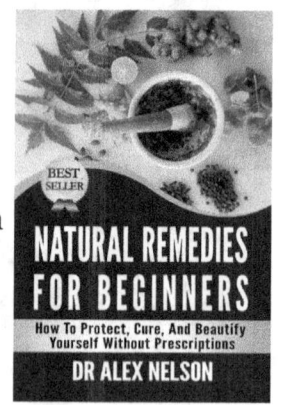

medical care these days, it is very expensive to get sick and we simply cannot afford to take a day off because of a cough or a cold.

Fortunately, the environment is so rich with resources that it actually offers us a less expensive alternative to synthetic medicine in the form of herbs, plants and oils.

This book will teach you that certain herbs and plants can cure certain ailments and how to aid illnesses the natural way. It also includes tips that you can easily follow at your home in order to keep yourself and your family members healthy, happy and free from diseases.